56 Cavity Preventing Juice Recipes:

Juice Your way to a Cavity-free Life

By

Joe Correa CSN

COPYRIGHT

This publication is designed to provide accurate and authoritative information in regard to the subject matter covered. It is sold with the understanding that neither the author nor the publisher is engaged in rendering medical advice. If medical advice or assistance is needed, consult with a doctor. This book is considered a guide and should not be used in any way detrimental to your health. Consult with a physician before starting this nutritional plan to make sure it's right for you.

ACKNOWLEDGEMENTS

This book is dedicated to my friends and family that have had mild or serious illnesses so that you may find a solution and make the necessary changes in your life.

56 Cavity Preventing Juice Recipes:

Juice Your way to a Cavity-free Life

By

Joe Correa CSN

CONTENTS

ABOUT THE AUTHOR

After years of Research, I honestly believe in the positive effects that proper nutrition can have over the body and mind. My knowledge and experience has helped me live healthier throughout the years and which I have shared with family and friends. The more you know about eating and drinking healthier, the sooner you will want to change your life and eating habits.

Nutrition is a key part in the process of being healthy and living longer so get started today. The first step is the most important and the most significant.

INTRODUCTION

56 Cavity Preventing Juice Recipes: Juice Your way to a Cavity-free Life

By Joe Correa CSN

A beautiful and radiant smile is one of the first things we notice in people. This is the basic physical characteristic which defines our character, our beauty, and self-confidence.

However, it's crucial to consider the medical issues related to poor tooth health. Bad oral hygiene and an unhealthy diet can lead to some serious problems like the increased risk of heart attack, stroke, diabetes, poor health in newborn babies, lung disease, weakened immune system, kidney and liver failure, and other diseases. From this, we can easily conclude that a healthy smile is a mirror of our overall health.

As they say "better safe than sorry". This is especially true when talking about oral health, especially if you keep in mind how little it takes to preserve healthy teeth, avoid complications, and prevent expensive dental procedures. The simplest and, at the same time, the healthiest method is to change your daily diet and have proper oral hygiene.

Proper oral hygiene is something we can all take care of on a daily basis. However, most of us fail to consider how proper nutrition and good eating habits and affect the long term health of our teeth. Large amounts of sugar, processed foods, and chemicals in our food, directly affect and damage teeth and lead to cavities.

This collection of powerful juices will be an excellent alternative to unhealthy snacks which are packed with sugar and cause the formation of cavities.

I went the step forward and tried out hundreds of juice combinations until I found these delicious recipes which will serve you well. These juices are full of antioxidants and different nutrients that will not only make your teeth stay healthy, but will also boost up your overall immune system and health.

This book will serve as your guide to a bright and healthy smile.

You're just a few minutes and a couple of ingredients away from these delicious and healthy juices.

56 CAVITY PREVENTING JUICE RECIPES: JUICE YOUR WAY TO A CAVITY-FREE LIFE

1.   Apple Spinach Juice

Ingredients:

1 large green apple, cored

1 cup of fresh mint, chopped

1 large orange, peeled

1 handful of fresh spinach, torn

3 oz of water

Preparation:

Wash the apple and remove the core. Cut into bite-sized pieces and set aside.

Peel the orange and divide into wedges. Set aside.

Combine mint and spinach in a colander and wash thoroughly under cold running water. Drain and torn with hands.

Now, combine apple, orange, mint, and spinach in a juicer and process until juiced. Transfer to serving glasses and then stir in the water.

Add some ice before serving and enjoy!

Nutritional information per serving: Kcal: 178, Protein: 4.4g, Carbs: 54.5g, Fats: 0.9g

2.   Cauliflower Cantaloupe Juice

Ingredients:

1 cup of cauliflower head

1 cup of cantaloupe, chopped

1 cup of fresh basil, chopped

1 cup of fresh kale, chopped

1 large cucumber

Preparation:

Trim off the outer leaves of cauliflower. Wash it and cut into small pieces. Fill the measuring cup and reserve the rest in the refrigerator.

Cut the cantaloupe in half. Scoop out the seeds and flesh. Cut two wedges and peel them. Chop into chunks and set aside. Reserve the rest of the cantaloupe in a refrigerator.

Combine basil and kale in a colander under cold running water. Drain and roughly chop it.

Wash the cucumber and cut into thick pieces. set aside.

Now, combine cauliflower, cantaloupe, basil, kale, and cucumber in a juicer and process until juiced. Transfer to serving glasses and add few ice cubes before serving.

Enjoy!

Nutritional information per serving: Kcal: 132, Protein: 8.9g, Carbs: 35.4g, Fats: 1.7g

3.   Avocado Lime Juice

Ingredients:

1 cup of avocado, chopped

1 large lime, peeled

1 large orange, peeled

1 large cucumber

2 oz of water

Preparation:

Peel the avocado and cut in half. Remove the pit and cut the avocado into small chunks. Fill the measuring cup and reserve the rest for some other juice.

Peel the orange and divide into wedges. Set aside.

Peel the lime and cut lengthwise in half. Set aside.

Wash the cucumber and cut into thick slices. Set aside.

Now, combine avocado, lime, orange, and cucumber in a juicer and process until juiced. Transfer to serving glasses and stir in the water.

Add some ice and serve immediately.

Nutritional information per serving: Kcal: 132, Protein: 8.9g, Carbs: 35.4g, Fats: 1.7g

4.   Sweet Pineapple Kiwi Juice

Ingredients:

1 cup of pineapple chunks

2 large kiwis, peeled

1 large lemon, peeled

1 large carrot

1 large yellow apple, cored

1 tbsp of liquid honey

Preparation:

Cut the top of a pineapple and peel it using a sharp knife. Cut into small chunks and fill the measuring cup. Reserve the rest of the pineapple in a refrigerator.

Peel the kiwis and lemon. Cut lengthwise in half and set aside.

Wash the carrot and cut into thick slices. Set aside.

Wash the apple and remove the core. Cut into bite-sized pieces and set aside.

Now, process pineapple, kiwis, lemon, carrot, and apple in a juicer. Transfer to serving glasses and stir in the liquid honey.

Add some ice before serving.

Nutritional information per serving: Kcal: 132, Protein: 8.9g, Carbs: 35.4g, Fats: 1.7g

5.   Spinach Squash Juice

Ingredients:

1 cup of butternut squash, cubed

1 cup of spinach, torn

1 large orange, peeled

1 large cucumber

1 ginger root slice, 1-inch

Preparation:

Peel the butternut squash and remove the seeds using a spoon. Cut into small cubes and reserve the rest of the squash for some other recipe. Wrap in a plastic foil and refrigerate.

Wash the spinach thoroughly under cold running water. Drain and torn with hands. Set aside.

Peel the orange and divide into wedges. Set aside.

Wash the cucumber and cut into thick slices. Set aside.

Peel the ginger root slice and set aside.

Now, combine squash, spinach, orange, cucumber, and ginger slice in a juicer and process until juiced.

Stir in some water to adjust the thickness if needed. Add some ice and serve immediately.

Enjoy!

Nutritional information per serving: Kcal: 209, Protein: 14.8g, Carbs: 61.6g, Fats: 2.1g

6.   Pumpkin Pie Juice

Ingredients:

2 cups of pumpkin, chopped

2 cups of cranberries

2 large oranges, peeled

¼ tsp of cinnamon, ground

¼ tsp of nutmeg, ground

2 oz of water

Preparation:

Peel the pumpkin and cut in half. Scoop out the seeds using a spoon. Cut two large wedges and peel them. Cut into small chunks and fill the measuring cups. Reserve the rest for later.

Place the cranberries in a colander and wash under cold running water. Drain and set aside.

Peel the oranges and divide into wedges. Set aside.

Now, combine pumpkin, cranberries, and oranges in a juicer and process until juiced. Transfer to serving glasses and stir in the cinnamon, nutmeg, and water.

Add some ice and serve immediately.

Nutritional information per serving: Kcal: 248, Protein: 6.6g, Carbs: 82.7g, Fats: 0.9g

7.   Red Lime Juice

Ingredients:

1 cup of beets, trimmed

3 large limes, peeled

1 cup of watercress

1 large green apple, cored

1 large cucumber

Preparation:

Wash the beets and trim off the green ends. Cut into bite-sized pieces and set aside.

Peel the limes and cut lengthwise in half. Set aside.

Wash the watercress thoroughly under cold running water. Drain and set aside.

Wash the apple and remove the core. Cut into bite-sized pieces. Set aside.

Wash the cucumber and cut into thick slices. Set aside.

Now, combine beets, limes, watercress, apple, and cucumber in a juicer and process until juiced.

Add some ice and serve.

Nutritional information per serving: Kcal: 211, Protein: 6.4g, Carbs: 63.5g, Fats: 1.1g

8.   Strawberry Cherry Juice

Ingredients:

1 cup of fresh strawberries, chopped

1 cup of fresh cherries, pitted

1 large lemon, peeled

1 tbsp of liquid honey

2 oz of water

Preparation:

Combine strawberries and cherries in a colander and wash under cold running water. Cut the strawberries into small pieces and set aside. Cut the cherries in half and remove the pits. Set aside.

Peel the lemon and cut lengthwise in half. Set aside.

Now, combine strawberries, cherries, and lemon in a juicer and process until juiced.

Transfer to serving glasses and stir in the liquid honey and water. Add some ice cubes before serving.

Enjoy!

Nutritional information per serving: Kcal: 195, Protein: 3.5g, Carbs: 59.8g, Fats: 1g

9.   Broccoli Orange Juice

Ingredients:

2 cups of broccoli, chopped

2 large oranges, peeled

1 small Fuji apple, cored

3 tbsp of fresh basil, torn

A handful of spinach

Preparation:

Wash the broccoli under cold running water and cut into small pieces. Set aside.

Peel the oranges and divide into wedges. Set aside.

Wash the apple and remove the core. Cut into bite-sized pieces and set aside.

Wash the basil and spinach thoroughly using a colander. Torn with hands and set aside.

Nutritional information per serving: Kcal: 195, Protein: 3.5g, Carbs: 43.8g, Fats: 1g

10.   Salted Vegetable Juice

Ingredients:

1 large tomato

1 large red bell pepper, chopped

1 cup of cucumber, chopped

1 spring onion, chopped

¼ tsp of Himalayan salt

3 oz of water

Preparation:

Place the tomato in a bowl and cut into quarters. Reserve the tomato juice while cutting and set aside.

Wash the bell pepper and cut in half. Remove the seeds and cut into small pieces. Set aside.

Wash the cucumber and cut into thick slices.

Wash the spring onion and chop it into small pieces. Set aside.

Now, combine tomato, bell pepper, cucumber, and onion in a juicer and process until juiced.

Transfer to a serving glasses and stir in the salt, water, and reserved tomato juice. Add some ice cubes before serving and enjoy!

Nutritional information per serving: Kcal: 73, Protein: 3.7g, Carbs: 20.1g, Fats: 0.9g

11.   Radish Leek Juice

Ingredients:

3 medium-sized radishes, trimmed

3 large leeks, chopped

1 large green apple, cored

1 cup of kale, torn

1 large cucumber

A handful of fresh spinach, torn

Preparation:

Wash the radishes and trim off the green ends. Cut into small pieces and set aside.

Wash the leeks and chop into small pieces. set aside.

Wash the apple and remove the core. Cut into bite-sized pieces and set aside.

Wash the cucumber and cut into thick slices. Set aside.

Combine kale and spinach in a colander. Wash thoroughly under cold running water and torn with hands.

Now, process radishes, leeks, apple, kale, cucumber, and spinach in a juicer. Transfer to serving glasses and add some ice before serving.

Enjoy!

Nutritional information per serving: Kcal: 315, Protein: 10.4g, Carbs: 85.3g, Fats: 2.2g

12.   Apricot Raspberry Juice

Ingredients:

1 cup of apricots, pitted and chopped

1 cup of raspberries

1 large lemon, peeled

1 cup of cucumber, chopped

1 medium-sized orange, peeled

2 oz of water

Preparation:

Wash the apricots and cut in half. Remove the pits and cut into bite-sized pieces. Fill the measuring cup and reserve the rest for some other juice.

Place the raspberries in a colander and wash thoroughly under cold running water. Drain and set aside.

Peel the lemon and cut lengthwise in half. Set aside.

Peel the orange and divide into wedges. Set aside.

Now, combine apricots, raspberries, lemon, and orange in a juicer and process until juiced.

Transfer to serving glasses and stir in the water. Add some ice and serve immediately.

Nutritional information per serving: Kcal: 166, Protein: 6g, Carbs: 55.7g, Fats: 1.8g

13. Crookneck Squash Asparagus Juice

Ingredients:

1 cup of fresh asparagus, trimmed

1 cup of crookneck squash, chopped

1 large honeydew melon wedge, peeled

1 large carrot

1 large kiwi, peeled

1 large cucumber

Preparation:

Wash the asparagus and trim off the woody ends. Cut into bite-sized pieces and set aside.

Wash the crookneck squash and cut in half. Scoop out the seeds using a spoon. Cut into small chunks and fill the measuring cup. Reserve the rest for another juice.

Cut the honeydew melon lengthwise in half. Scoop out the seeds using a spoon. Cut one large wedge and peel it. Cut into small chunks and fill the measuring cup. Wrap the rest of the melon in a plastic foil and refrigerate.

Peel the kiwi and cut lengthwise in half. Set aside.

Wash the carrot and cucumber and cut into thick slices. Set aside.

Now, process asparagus, crookneck squash, honeydew melon, carrot, kiwi, and cucumber in a juicer.

Transfer to serving glasses and add some ice before serving.

Enjoy!

Nutritional information per serving: Kcal: 183, Protein: 8.5g, Carbs: 52.6g, Fats: 1.6g

14.   Kiwi Zucchini Juice

Ingredients:

3 large kiwis, peeled

1 large zucchini, seeded

1 large lime, peeled

1 cup of pomegranate seeds

1 large orange, peeled

Preparation:

Peel the kiwis and cut lengthwise in half. Set aside.

Wash the zucchini and cut in half. Scoop out the seeds using a spoon. Cut into small chunks and set aside.

Peel the lime and cut lengthwise in half. Set aside.

Cut the top of the pomegranate fruit using a sharp knife. Slice down to each of the white membranes inside of the fruit. Pop the seeds into a measuring cup and set aside.

Peel the orange and divide into wedges. Set aside.

Now, process kiwis, zucchini, lime, pomegranate seeds, and orange in a juicer.

Transfer to a serving glasses and add some ice cubes before serving.

Nutritional information per serving: Kcal: 183, Protein: 8.5g, Carbs: 52.6g, Fats: 1.6g

15.   Peppermint Juice

Ingredients:

2 large lemons, peeled

1 large lime, peeled

2 large oranges, peeled

1 cup of fresh mint, torn

¼ tsp of pure peppermint extract

Preparation:

Peel the lemons and lime. Cut lengthwise in half and set aside.

Peel the orange and divide into wedges. Set aside.

Place the mint in a colander and wash thoroughly under cold running water. Drain and torn with hands. Set aside.

Nutritional information per serving: Kcal: 178, Protein: 5.8g, Carbs: 61.5g, Fats: 1.1g

16.   Mango Blueberry Juice

Ingredients:

1 cup of mango chunks

1 cup of blueberries

1 large cucumber

1 medium-sized green apple, cored

2 oz of water

Preparation:

Wash the mango and cut into chunks. Fill the measuring cup and reserve the rest for some other juice. Set aside.

Place the blueberries in a colander and wash under cold running water. Drain and set aside.

Wash the apple and remove the core. Cut into bite-sized pieces and set aside.

Now, combine mango, blueberries, and apple in a juicer and process until juiced.

Transfer to serving glasses and stir in the water. Add some ice before serving and enjoy!

Nutritional information per serving: Kcal: 178, Protein: 5.8g, Carbs: 61.5g, Fats: 1.1g

17.   Vanilla Melon Juice

Ingredients:

1 cup of watermelon, seeded

1 cup of cantaloupe, seeded

1 large green apple, cored

1 medium-sized banana

¼ tsp of vanilla extract

2 oz of water

Preparation:

Cut the watermelon lengthwise. For one cup, you will need about one large wedge. Peel and cut into chunks. Remove the seeds and set aside. Reserve the rest of the melon for some other juices.

Cut the cantaloupe in half. Scoop out the seeds and flesh. Cut two wedges and peel them. Chop into chunks and set aside. Reserve the rest of the cantaloupe in a refrigerator.

Wash the apple and remove the core. Cut into bite-sized pieces and set aside.

Peel the banana and chop into small chunks. Set aside.

Now, combine watermelon, cantaloupe, apple, and banana in a juicer and process until juiced.

Transfer to serving glasses and stir in the vanilla extract and water. Add some ice and serve immediately.

Enjoy!

Nutritional information per serving: Kcal: 294, Protein: 4.6g, Carbs: 83.3g, Fats: 1.3g

18.   Carrot Lettuce Juice

Ingredients:

4 large carrots

1 cup of red leaf lettuce, torn

1 large lemon, peeled

1 large red apple, cored

Preparation:

Wash the carrots and cut into thick slices. Set aside.

Wash the lettuce thoroughly under cold running water. Torn with hands and set aside.

Peel the lemon and cut lengthwise in half. Set aside.

Wash the apple and remove the core. Cut into bite-sized pieces and set aside.

Now, process carrots, lettuce, lemon, and apple in a juicer. Transfer to serving glasses and add some ice before serving.

Enjoy!

Nutritional information per serving: Kcal: 231, Protein: 4.4g, Carbs: 70g, Fats: 1.4g

19.   Spicy Tomato Juice

Ingredients:

2 large Roma tomatoes

1 large celery stalk

1 cup of cucumber, sliced

¼ tsp of Himalayan salt

¼ tsp of black pepper, ground

¼ tsp of Cayenne pepper, ground

Preparation:

Place the tomato in a medium bowl. Cut into quarters and reserve the tomato juice while cutting. Set aside.

Wash the celery and cut into small pieces and set aside.

Wash the cucumber and cut into thick slices. Set aside.

Now, combine tomato, celery, and cucumber in a juicer and process until juiced.

Transfer to serving glasses and stir in the salt, pepper, and Cayenne pepper.

Add some ice before serving and enjoy!

Nutritional information per serving: Kcal: 61, Protein: 3.9g, Carbs: 17.9g, Fats: 0.9g

20.   Artichoke Protein Juice

Ingredients:

1 large artichoke head

1 large lime, peeled

1 cup of kale, torn

1 large cucumber

A handful of spinach, torn

Preparation:

Trim off the outer leaves of the artichoke using a sharp knife. Cut into small pieces and set aside.

Peel the lime and cut lengthwise in half. Set aside.

Wash the kale and spinach thoroughly under cold running water. Drain and torn with hands. Set aside.

Wash the cucumber and cut into thick slices. Set aside.

Now, combine artichoke, lime, kale, cucumber, and spinach in a juicer and process until juiced.

Transfer to serving glasses and add some ice before serving.

Enjoy!

Nutritional information per serving: Kcal: 117, Protein: 11.1g, Carbs: 38.6g, Fats: 1.3g

21. Salted Bell Pepper Juice

Ingredients:

1 large red bell pepper, seeded

1 large green bell pepper, seeded

1 large fennel bulb

1 large carrot

1 cup of Swiss chards, chopped

¼ tsp of Cayenne pepper, ground

¼ tsp of salt

Preparation:

Wash the bell peppers and cut in half. Remove the seeds and cut into small slices. Set aside.

Wash the fennel bulb and trim off the wilted outer layers. Cut into small chunks and set aside.

Wash the carrot and cut into thick slices. Set aside.

Wash the Swiss chard thoroughly under cold running water. Drain and roughly chop it. Fill the measuring cup and reserve the rest for some other juice. Set aside.

Now, combine bell peppers, fennel, carrot, and Swiss chards in a juicer and process until juiced. Transfer to serving glasses and add some ice cubes before serving.

Nutritional information per serving: Kcal: 130, Protein: 7.2g, Carbs: 42.8g, Fats: 1.4g

22.   Sweet Blueberry Juice

Ingredients:

1 cup of blueberries

1 large lemon, peeled

1 large orange, peeled

1 large green apple, cored

1 tbsp of liquid honey

Preparation:

Place the blueberries in a colander and wash under cold running water. Drain and set aside.

Peel the lemon and cut lengthwise in half. Set aside.

Peel the orange and divide into wedges. Set aside.

Wash the apple and remove the core. Cut into bite-sized pieces and set aside.

Now, combine blueberries, lemon, orange, and apple in a juicer and process until juiced.

Transfer to serving glasses and stir in the liquid honey.

Add few ice cubes or refrigerate before serving

Nutritional information per serving: Kcal: 305, Protein: 4.3g, Carbs: 76.5g, Fats: 1.3g

23.   Kale Leek Juice

Ingredients:

3 cups of kale, chopped

3 large leeks

1 cup of broccoli, chopped

1 large cucumber

1 small ginger root slice, 1-inch

Preparation:

Wash the kale thoroughly under cold running water using a colander. Drain and torn roughly chop it. Set aside.

Wash the leeks and cut into small pieces. Set aside.

Wash the broccoli and cut into bite-sized pieces. Fill the measuring cup and reserve the rest for some other juice.

Wash the cucumber and cut into thick slices. Set aside.

Peel the ginger root slice and set aside.

Now, process kale, leeks, broccoli, cucumber and ginger in a juicer.

Transfer to serving glasses and refrigerate for 30 minutes before serving.

Nutritional information per serving: Kcal: 275, Protein: 17.2g, Carbs: 72.7g, Fats: 3.3g

24.   Beet Pomegranate Juice

Ingredients:

2 large beets, trimmed

1 cup of pomegranate seeds

1 large cucumber

1 small ginger root knob, 1-inch

2 oz of water

Preparation:

Wash the beets and trim off the green ends. Cut into small pieces and set aside.

Cut the top of the pomegranate fruit using a sharp knife. Slice down to each of the white membranes inside of the fruit. Pop the seeds into a measuring cup and set aside.

Wash the cucumber and cut into thick slices. Set aside.

Peel the ginger knob and set aside.

Now, process beets, pomegranate seeds, cucumber, and ginger in a juicer.

Transfer to serving glasses and add some ice cubes or refrigerate before serving.

Nutritional information per serving: Kcal: 180, Protein: 7.4g, Carbs: 51.7g, Fats: 1.8g

25.   Pineapple Honey Juice

Ingredients:

1 cup of pineapple, chopped

1 cup of apricots, pitted and halved

1 large cucumber

1 tbsp of liquid honey

2 oz of water

Preparation:

Cut the top of a pineapple and peel it using a sharp knife. Cut into small chunks and fill the measuring cup. Reserve the rest of the pineapple in a refrigerator.

Wash the apricots and cut in half. Remove the pits and cut into bite-sized pieces. Fill the measuring cup and reserve the rest for some other juice.

Wash the cucumber and cut into thick slices. Set aside.

Now, combine pineapple, apricots, and cucumber in a juicer and process until juiced.

Transfer to serving glasses and stir in the liquid honey and water.

Add some ice before serving and enjoy!

Nutritional information per serving: Kcal: 234, Protein: 5g, Carbs: 49.8g, Fats: 1.1g

26.   Honeydew Melon Juice

Ingredients:

2 large honeydew melon wedges

1 large lemon, peeled

1 large green apple, cored

1 medium-sized orange, peeled

2 oz of water

Preparation:

Cut the honeydew melon lengthwise in half. Scoop out the seeds using a spoon. Cut two large wedges and peel them. Cut into small chunks and fill the measuring cup. Wrap the rest of the melon in a plastic foil and refrigerate.

Peel the lemon and cut lengthwise in half. Set aside.

Wash the apple and remove the core. Cut into bite-sized pieces and set aside.

Peel the orange and divide into wedges. Set aside.

Now, combine honeydew melon, lemon, apple, and orange in a juicer and process until juiced. Transfer to serving glasses and add some ice before serving.

Enjoy!

Nutritional information per serving: Kcal: 263, Protein: 4.5g, Carbs: 77.9g, Fats: 1.1g

27.   Leek Asparagus Juice

Ingredients:

2 large leeks

1 cup of asparagus, trimmed

1 cup of yellow pumpkin, chopped

1 cup of Romaine lettuce, chopped

2 tbsp of fresh parsley, chopped

1 large cucumber

Preparation:

Wash the leeks and chop into small pieces. Set aside.

Wash the asparagus and trim off the woody ends. Chop into small pieces and set aside.

Peel the pumpkin and cut in half. Scoop out the seeds using a spoon. Cut one large wedge and peel it. Cut into small chunks and fill the measuring cup. Reserve the rest for some other juice.

Combine lettuce and parsley in a colander and wash thoroughly under cold running water. Drain and roughly chop it.

Wash the cucumber and cut into thick slices. Set aside.

Now, process leeks, asparagus, pumpkin, lettuce, parsley, and cucumber in a juicer. Transfer to serving glasses and add some ice, or refrigerate for 20 minutes before serving.

Nutritional information per serving: Kcal: 185, Protein: 9.5g, Carbs: 50.8g, Fats: 1.3g

28.   Sweet Potato Turmeric Juice

Ingredients:

1 cup of sweet potato, chopped

2 large carrots

1 small cauliflower head

¼ tsp of turmeric, ground

¼ tsp of Himalayan salt

3 oz of water

Preparation:

Peel the sweet potato and cut it into bite-sized pieces. Fill the measuring cup and reserve the rest for some other juice.

Wash the carrots and cut into thin slices. Set aside.

Trim off the outer leaves of cauliflower. Wash it and cut into small pieces. Set aside.

Now, combine sweet potato, carrots, and cauliflower in a juicer and process until juiced.

Transfer to serving glasses and stir in the turmeric, salt, and water.

Refrigerate for 30 minutes before serving.

Nutritional information per serving: Kcal: 187, Protein: 8.5g, Carbs: 53.7g, Fats: 1.1g

29.   Vanilla Strawberry Juice

Ingredients:

1 cup of strawberries, halved

1 large orange, peeled

1 small green apple, cored

3 oz of coconut water

¼ tsp of vanilla extract

Preparation:

Place the strawberries in a colander and wash under cold running water. Drain and cut in half. Set aside.

Peel the orange and divide into wedges. Set aside.

Wash the apple and remove the core. Cut into bite-sized pieces and set aside.

Now, combine strawberries, orange, and apple in a juicer and process until juiced.

Transfer to serving glasses and add some ice before serving.

Enjoy!

Nutritional information per serving: Kcal: 211, Protein: 3.5g, Carbs: 58g, Fats: 0.9g

30.   Summer Tropical Juice

Ingredients:

1 cup of papaya, chopped

1 cup of mango, chopped

1 large orange, peeled

1 large lime, peeled

3 oz of coconut water

1 tbsp of honey

Preparation:

Peel the papaya and cut lengthwise in half. Scoop out the black seeds using a spoon. Cut into small chunks and fill the measuring cup. Reserve the rest for some other juice.

Wash the mango and chop into chunks. Set aside.

Peel the orange and divide into wedges. Set aside.

Peel the lime and cut lengthwise in half. Set aside.

Now, combine papaya, mango, orange, and lime in a juicer and process until juiced.

Transfer to serving glasses and stir in the coconut water and honey. Add some ice before serving and enjoy!

Nutritional information per serving: Kcal: 295, Protein: 3.9g, Carbs: 75g, Fats: 1.2g

31. Swiss Chard Kale Juice

Ingredients:

2 cups of Swiss chards, torn

1 cup of kale, torn

1 large lime, peeled

1 large cucumber

1 cup of beet greens, chopped

1 cup of Romaine lettuce, chopped

¼ tsp of Himalayan salt

Preparation:

Combine Swiss chards, lettuce, and kale in a colander and wash thoroughly under cold running water. Drain and torn with hands. Set aside.

Peel the lime and cut lengthwise in half. Set aside.

Wash the cucumber and cut into thick slices. Set aside.

Wash the beet greens thoroughly and roughly chop it. Fill the measuring cup and reserve the rest for some other juice.

Now, combine Swiss chards, lettuce, kale, lime, cucumber, and beet greens in a juicer and process until juiced.

Transfer to serving glasses and stir in the salt. Add some ice and serve immediately.

Nutritional information per serving: Kcal: 88, Protein: 7.7g, Carbs: 26.3g, Fats: 1.3g

32. Honeycrisp Plum Juice

Ingredients:

3 large plums, pitted

1 large Honeycrisp apple, cored

1 large orange, peeled

1 small ginger root slice, 1-inch

2 oz of water

Preparation:

Wash the plums and cut in half. Remove the pits and cut into small pieces. Set aside.

Wash the apple and remove the core. Cut into bite-sized pieces and set aside.

Peel the orange and divide into wedges. Set aside.

Peel the ginger root and set aside.

Now, combine plums, apple, orange, and ginger in a juicer and process until juiced. Transfer to serving glasses and add some ice before serving.

Enjoy!

Nutritional information per serving: Kcal: 88, Protein: 7.7g, Carbs: 26.3g, Fats: 1.3g

33. Collard Greens Broccoli Juice

Ingredients:

2 cups of collard greens, chopped

2 cups of broccoli, chopped

1 cup of fresh basil, chopped

1 large cucumber

¼ tsp of Himalayan salt

2 oz of water

Preparation:

Combine collard greens and basil in a colander. Wash thoroughly under cold running water and drain. Roughly chop and set aside.

Wash the broccoli and chop into bite-sized pieces. Set aside.

Wash the cucumber and cut into thick slices. Set aside.

Now, combine collard greens, basil, broccoli, and cucumber in a juicer and process until juiced. Transfer to serving glasses and add some ice before serving.

Enjoy!

Nutritional information per serving: Kcal: 97, Protein: 10.1g, Carbs: 27.5g, Fats: 1.6g

34.   Blackberry Kiwi Juice

Ingredients:

2 cups of blackberries

2 large kiwis, peeled

1 large Fuji apple, cored

1 cup of watermelon, seeded

2 oz of coconut water

Preparation:

Wash the blueberries under cold running water using a colander. Drain and set aside.

Peel the kiwis and cut lengthwise in half. Set aside.

Wash the apple and remove the core. Cut into bite-sized pieces and set aside.

Cut the watermelon in half. Cut one large wedge and peel it. Chop into small chunks and remove the seeds. Fill the measuring cup and refrigerate the rest for some other juice.

Now, combine blueberries, kiwis, apple, and watermelon in a juicer and process until juiced. Transfer to serving glasses and stir in coconut water.

Add some ice and serve immediately.

Nutritional information per serving: Kcal: 315, Protein: 7.2g, Carbs: 97.9g, Fats: 2.8g

35. Salted Radish Arugula Juice

Ingredients:

5 large radishes, trimmed

1 cup of arugula, torn

1 large leek, chopped

1 large green bell pepper, seeded

1 large cucumber

¼ tsp of Himalayan salt

Preparation:

Wash the radishes and trim off the green parts. Cut into bite-sized pieces and set aside.

Wash the arugula thoroughly under cold running water and torn with hands. Set aside.

Wash the leek and cut into small pieces. Set aside.

Wash the bell pepper and cut in half. Remove the seeds and chop into small pieces. Set aside.

Wash the cucumber and cut into thick pieces. Set aside.

Now, process radishes, arugula, leek, bell pepper, and cucumber in a juicer. Transfer to serving glasses and stir in the salt. Refrigerate for 20 minutes before serving.

Nutritional information per serving: Kcal: 130, Protein: 7.9g, Carbs: 37.8g, Fats: 1.1g

36. Citrus Avocado Juice

Ingredients:

1 cup of avocado chunks

1 large cucumber

1 large lime, peeled

1 large lemon, peeled

2 oz of water

Preparation:

Peel the avocado and cut in half. Remove the pit and cut into chunks. Fill the measuring cup and reserve the rest for some other juice.

Wash the cucumber and cut into thick slices. Set aside.

Peel the lime and lemon. Cut lengthwise in half and set aside.

Now, combine avocado, cucumber, lime, and lemon in a juicer and process until juiced.

Transfer to a serving glasses and stir in the water. Add some ice before serving or refrigerate for 30 minutes before serving.

Enjoy!

Nutritional information per serving: Kcal: 260, Protein: 5.8g, Carbs: 32.8g, Fats: 22.5g

37.   Red Grape Cherry Juice

Ingredients:

2 cups of red grapes

1 cup of cherries, pitted

1 medium-sized Fuji apple, cored

2 tbsp of fresh mint, chopped

1 tbsp of liquid honey

2 oz of water

Preparation:

Combine grapes and cherries in a large colander. Wash under cold running water and drain. Cut the cherries in half and remove the pits. Set aside.

Wash the apple and remove the core. Cut into bite-sized pieces and set aside.

Wash the mint and roughly chop it. Set aside.

Now, combine grapes, cherries, apple, and mint in a juicer and process until juiced.

Transfer to serving glasses and add some ice before serving.

Nutritional information per serving: Kcal: 369, Protein: 3.5g, Carbs: 104g, Fats: 1.4g

38.   Ginger Peach Juice

Ingredients:

2 large peaches, pitted and chopped

1 medium-sized Honeycrisp apple, cored

1 large orange, peeled

1 small ginger root slice, 1-inch

1 tbsp of honey

2 oz of water

Preparation:

Wash the peaches and cut in half. Remove the pits and cut into small pieces.

Wash the apple and remove the core. Cut into bite-sized pieces and set aside.

Peel the orange and divide into wedges. Set aside.

Peel the ginger root slice and set aside.

Now, process peaches, apple, orange, and ginger in a juicer.

Transfer to serving glasses and stir in the honey and water.

Add a few ice cubes before serving and enjoy!

Nutritional information per serving: Kcal: 323, Protein: 5.6g, Carbs: 97.4g, Fats: 1.4g

39. Zucchini Carrot Juice

Ingredients:

2 large zucchini, chopped

1 large carrot

1 cup of purple cabbage, chopped

1 large red bell pepper, seeded

¼ tsp of Himalayan salt

Preparation:

Peel the zucchinis and cut in half. Scrape out the seeds and cut into small chunks. Set aside.

Wash the carrot and cut into thick slices. Set aside.

Wash the cabbage thoroughly under cold running water and roughly chop it. Fill the measuring cup and reserve the rest for some other juice.

Wash the bell pepper and cut in half. Remove the seeds and chop into small slices.

Now, combine zucchini, carrot, cabbage, and bell pepper in a juicer and process until juiced.

Add some ice cubes before serving and enjoy.

Nutritional information per serving: Kcal: 163, Protein: 11.4g, Carbs: 43.4g, Fats: 2.8g

40.   Cherry Tomato Rosemary Juice

Ingredients:

1 cup of cherry tomatoes

2 cups of beet greens

1 large red bell pepper, seeded

1 cup of celery, chopped

1 small rosemary sprig

Preparation:

Wash the cherry tomatoes and place them in a bowl. Cut in half and fill the measuring cup. Reserve the tomato juice while cutting. Set aside.

Combine beet greens and celery in a colander and wash thoroughly under cold running water. Roughly chop it and set aside.

Wash the bell pepper and cut in half. remove the seeds and chop into small pieces. Set aside.

Now, combine cherry tomatoes, beet greens, bell pepper, and celery in a juicer and process until juiced.

Transfer to serving glasses and stir in the reserved tomato juice and sprinkle with some rosemary for some extra flavor.

Enjoy!

Nutritional information per serving: Kcal: 71, Protein: 5.5g, Carbs: 22.8g, Fats: 1.1g

41.   Grapefruit Mango Juice

Ingredients:

1 large grapefruit

1 cup of mango chunks

1 small Granny Smith apple, cored

1 large lemon, peeled

1 small ginger root slice, 1-inch

3 oz of coconut water

Preparation:

Peel the grapefruit and divide into wedges. Set aside.

Wash the mango and cut into chunks. Fill the measuring cup and reserve the rest for some other juice.

Wash the apple and remove the core. Cut into bite-sized pieces and set aside.

Peel the lemon and cut lengthwise in half. Set aside.

Peel the ginger root slice and set aside.

Now, process grapefruit, mango, apple, lemon, and ginger in a juicer. Transfer to serving glasses and stir in the coconut water.

Refrigerate for 20 minutes before serving.

Nutritional information per serving: Kcal: 71, Protein: 5.5g, Carbs: 22.8g, Fats: 1.1g

42. Dark Green Juice

Ingredients:

1 large fennel bulb

1 large artichoke head

1 cup of kale, chopped

1 cup of asparagus, trimmed

1 cup of Brussel sprouts, trimmed

1 cup of Swiss chard, chopped

¼ tsp of Cayenne pepper, ground

Preparation:

Wash the fennel bulb and trim off the wilted outer layers. Cut into small chunks and set aside.

Trim off the outer leaves of the artichoke. Wash it and cut into bite-sized pieces. Set aside.

Combine kale and Swiss chard in a colander and wash under cold running water. Roughly chop it and set aside.

Wash the asparagus and trim off the woody ends. Cut into small pieces and set aside.

Wash the Brussel sprouts and trim off the outer layers. Cut in half and set aside.

Now, process fennel, artichoke, kale, asparagus, Brussel sprouts, and Swiss chard in a juicer. Transfer to serving glasses and stir in the Cayenne pepper.

Refrigerate for 15 minutes before serving.

Nutritional information per serving: Kcal: 154, Protein: 17.6g, Carbs: 54.4g, Fats: 1.8g

43. Turnip Greens Zucchini Juice

Ingredients:

1 cup of turnip greens

1 large zucchini, chopped

1 cup of mustard greens, chopped

1 cup of fresh basil, chopped

1 large cucumber

A handful of spinach

Preparation:

Wash the turnip greens thoroughly and roughly chop it into. Fill the measuring cup and reserve the rest for some other juice.

Peel the zucchini and cut in half. Scrape out the seeds using a spoon. Cut into small chunks and set aside.

Combine mustard greens, basil, and spinach in a colander. Wash thoroughly under cold running water and roughly chop it. Set aside.

Wash the cucumber and cut into thick slices. Set aside.

Now, process turnip greens, zucchini, mustard greens, basil, cucumber, and spinach in a juicer.

Transfer to serving glasses and add few ice cubes before serving.

Enjoy!

Nutritional information per serving: Kcal: 154, Protein: 17.6g, Carbs: 54.4g, Fats: 1.8g

44.   Cantaloupe Cranberry Juice

Ingredients:

1 cup of cantaloupe, chopped

1 cup of cranberries

1 cup of watermelon, seeded

1 large lemon, peeled

1 small Ginger Gold apple, cored

1 small ginger root slice

Preparation:

Cut the cantaloupe in half. Scoop out the seeds and flesh. Cut two wedges and peel them. Chop into chunks and fill the measuring cup. Reserve the rest of the cantaloupe in a refrigerator.

Wash the cranberries under cold running water using a colander. Drain and set aside.

Cut the watermelon lengthwise in half. For one cup, you will need about 1 large wedge. Peel and cut into chunks. Remove the seeds and set aside.

Peel the lemon and cut lengthwise in half. Set aside.

Wash the apple and remove the core. Cut into bite-sized pieces and set aside.

Peel the ginger root and set aside.

Now, combine cantaloupe, cranberries, watermelon, lemon, apple, and ginger in a juicer and process until juiced.

Transfer to serving glasses and add some ice before serving.

Nutritional information per serving: Kcal: 194, Protein: 3.6g, Carbs: 59.7g, Fats: 1.1g

45.   Lime Guava Juice

Ingredients:

1 large lime, peeled

1 large guava, chopped

1 large orange, peeled

1 medium-sized apple, cored

3 oz of water

Preparation:

Peel the lime and cut lengthwise in half. Set aside.

Peel and wash the guava. Cut into small chunks and set aside.

Peel the orange and divide into wedges. Set aside.

Wash the apple and remove the core. Cut into bite-sized pieces and set aside.

Now, combine lime, guava, orange, and apple in a juicer and process until juiced.

Transfer to serving glasses and stir in the water. Add some ice and serve immediately.

Nutritional information per serving: Kcal: 163, Protein: 3.5g, Carbs: 49.7g, Fats: 1g

46.   Beets Romaine Juice

Ingredients:

2 cups of beets, trimmed

1 cup of Romaine lettuce, chopped

1 cup of celery, chopped

1 cup of watercress, chopped

1 cup of basil, chopped

A handful of spinach

¼ tsp of Himalayan salt

2 oz of water

Preparation:

Wash the beets and trim off the green parts. Cut into bite-sized pieces and set aside.

Combine lettuce, celery, watercress, basil, and spinach in a colander. Wash thoroughly under cold running water and drain. Roughly chop and set aside.

Now, process beets, lettuce, celery, watercress, basil, and spinach in a juicer.

Transfer to serving glasses and stir in the salt and water. Add few ice cubes before serving and enjoy!

Nutritional information per serving: Kcal: 111, Protein: 8.1g, Carbs: 32.7g, Fats: 1.1g

47.   Raspberry Peach Juice

Ingredients:

1 cup of raspberries

1 large peach, pitted and halved

1 large green apple, cored

1 cup of cantaloupe, chopped

1 small ginger root slice, 1-inch

1 tbsp of liquid honey

Preparation:

Wash the raspberries under cold running water using a colander. Drain and set aside.

Wash the peach and cut in half. Remove the pit and cut into small pieces. Set aside.

Wash the apple and remove the core. Cut into bite-sized pieces and set aside.

Cut the cantaloupe in half. Scoop out the seeds and flesh. Cut two wedges and peel them. Chop into chunks and fill the measuring cup. Reserve the rest of the cantaloupe in a refrigerator.

Peel the ginger root slice and set aside.

Now, combine raspberries, peach, apple, cantaloupe, and ginger in a juicer and process until juiced.

Add some ice or refrigerate before serving.

Nutritional information per serving: Kcal: 295, Protein: 5.3g, Carbs: 89.5g, Fats: 1.9g

48.   Carrot Agave Juice

Ingredients:

3 large carrots

1 cup of beets, trimmed and chopped

1 large cucumber

1 large orange, peeled

2 oz of water

½ tsp of agave nectar

Preparation:

Wash the carrots and cut into thick slices. Set aside.

Wash the beets and trim off the green parts. Cut into bite-sized pieces and fill the measuring cup. Reserve the rest for some other juice.

Wash the cucumber and cut into thick slices. Set aside.

Peel the orange and divide into wedges. Set aside.

Now, combine carrots, beets, cucumber, and orange in a juicer and process until juiced.

Transfer to serving glasses and stir in the water and agave nectar. Add some ice and serve immediately.

Nutritional information per serving: Kcal: 296, Protein: 7.9g, Carbs: 86.2g, Fats: 1.3g

49.   Spicy Fennel Juice

Ingredients:

1 large fennel bulb

1 cup of mustard greens

1 cup of kale, chopped

2 large radishes, chopped

1 cup of parsley, chopped

1 large cucumber

¼ tsp of Cayenne pepper, ground

¼ tsp of Himalayan salt

2 oz of water

Preparation:

Wash the fennel bulb and trim off the wilted outer layers. Cut into small chunks and set aside.

Combine mustard greens, kale, and parsley in a colander. Wash thoroughly under cold running water. Drain and roughly chop it. Set aside.

Wash the radishes and trim off the green parts. Cut into bite-sized pieces and set aside.

Wash the cucumber and cut into thick slices. Set aside.

Now, combine fennel, mustard greens, kale, parsley, and radishes in a juicer and process until juiced.

Transfer to serving glasses and stir in the Cayenne pepper and water. You can add some salt but this is optional.

Refrigerate for 30 minutes before serving.

Nutritional information per serving: Kcal: 130, Protein: 11.2g, Carbs: 40.9g, Fats: 2.1g

50.   Peach Pomegranate Juice

Ingredients:

1 large peach, pitted and halved

1 large lemon, peeled

1 large orange, peeled

1 large lime, peeled

1 cup of pomegranate seeds

3 oz of water

1 tbsp of honey

Preparation:

Wash the peach and cut in half. Remove the pit and cut into small pieces. Set aside.

Peel the lemon and lime. Cut lengthwise in half and set aside.

Peel the orange and divide into wedges. Set aside.

Cut the top of the pomegranate fruit using a sharp knife. Slice down to each of the white membranes inside of the fruit. Pop the seeds into measuring cup and set aside.

Now, combine peach, lemon, orange, lime, and pomegranate seeds in a juicer and process until juiced.

Transfer to serving glasses and stir in the water and honey. Add some ice and serve!

Nutritional information per serving: Kcal: 265, Protein: 5.6g, Carbs: 63.7g, Fats: 1.8g

51.   Protein Brussel Sprout Juice

Ingredients:

2 cups of Brussel sprouts, trimmed and halved

1 large cucumber

1 cup of Romaine lettuce, chopped

1 large leek, chopped

1 large bunch of spinach

¼ tsp of Himalayan salt

2 oz f water

Preparation:

Trim off the outer leaves of the Brussel sprouts. Wash and cut in half. Set aside.

Wash the cucumber and cut into thick slices. Set aside.

Combine lettuce, leek, and spinach in a colander. Wash under cold running water. Drain and roughly chop it. Set aside.

Now, process Brussel sprouts, cucumber, lettuce, leek, and spinach in a juicer.

Transfer to serving glasses and stir in some water. Add some ice and serve immediately.

Nutritional information per serving: Kcal: 189, Protein: 19.5g, Carbs: 53.1g, Fats: 2.6g

52.   Plum Tomato Juice

Ingredients:

1 cup of plum tomatoes

1 cup of basil, torn

1 large red bell pepper, seeded

1 large lemon, peeled

1 rosemary sprig

¼ tsp of Himalayan salt

Preparation:

Wash the plum tomatoes and place in a bowl. Cut in half and reserve the juice while cutting. Set aside.

Wash the basil thoroughly under cold running water using a colander. Drain and torn with hands. Set aside.

Wash the bell pepper and cut in half. Remove the seeds and cut into small pieces. Set aside.

Peel the lemon and cut lengthwise in half. Set aside.

Now, combine tomatoes, basil, pepper, and lemon in a juicer and process until juiced. Transfer to serving glasses and stir in the salt. Sprinkle with some rosemary for some extra taste.

Refrigerate for 30 minutes before serving.

Nutritional information per serving: Kcal: 189, Protein: 19.5g, Carbs: 53.1g, Fats: 2.6g

53.   Sweet Potato Pumpkin Juice

Ingredients:

1 cup of pumpkin, chopped

1 cup of sweet potato, chopped

1 large carrot

1 large cucumber

1 medium-sized zucchini, chopped

¼ tsp of Himalayan salt

¼ tsp of ginger, ground

Preparation:

Peel the pumpkin and cut in half. Scoop out the seeds using a spoon. Cut one large wedge and peel it. Cut into small chunks and fill the measuring cup. Reserve the rest for later.

Peel the sweet potato and cut into small chunks. Set aside.

Wash the carrot and cut into thick slices. Set aside.

Peel the zucchini and cut in half. Scrape out the seeds using a spoon. Cut into bite-sized pieces and set aside.

Wash the cucumber and cut into thick slices. Set aside.

Now, combine pumpkin, potato, carrot, cucumber, and zucchini in a juicer and process until juiced.

Transfer to serving glasses and stir in the salt and ginger. Add some water to adjust the thickness of the juice.

Add some ice and serve.

Nutritional information per serving: Kcal: 214, Protein: 8.3g, Carbs: 58.6g, Fats: 1.3g

54.   Sweet Melon Juice

Ingredients:

1 large honeydew melon wedge

1 cup of watermelon, seeded

1 large lemon, peeled

1 large green apple, cored

1 tbsp of liquid honey

2 oz of water

Preparation:

Cut the honeydew melon lengthwise in half. Scoop out the seeds using a spoon. Cut one large wedge and peel it. Cut into small chunks and set aside. Wrap the rest of the melon in a plastic foil and refrigerate.

Cut the watermelon lengthwise. For one cup, you will need about 1 large wedge. Peel and cut into chunks. Remove the seeds and set aside. Reserve the rest for some other juice.

Peel the lemon and cut lengthwise in half. Set aside.

Wash the apple and remove the core. Cut into bite-sized pieces and set aside.

Now, combine honeydew melon, watermelon, lemon, and apple in a juicer and process until juiced.

Transfer to serving glasses and stir in the honey and water. Add few ice cubes or refrigerate for 20 minutes before serving.

Enjoy!

Nutritional information per serving: Kcal: 264, Protein: 3.3g, Carbs: 76.4g, Fats: 1g

55.　Asparagus Parsnip Juice

Ingredients:

1 cup of asparagus, trimmed and chopped

1 cup of parsnip, chopped

1 cup of turnip greens, chopped

1 large leek, chopped

1 cup of fresh mint, chopped

1 large cucumber

2 oz of water

Preparation:

Wash the asparagus and trim off the green ends. Cut into small pieces and set aside.

Wash the parsnip and cut into thick slices. Fill the measuring cup and reserve the rest for some other juice.

Combine turnip greens, leek, and mint in a colander and wash thoroughly under cold running water. Roughly chop all and set aside.

Wash the cucumber and cut into thick slices. Set aside.

Now, combine asparagus, parsnip, turnip greens, leek, mint, and cucumber in a juicer and process until juiced.

Transfer to serving glasses and stir in the water. Add some ice and serve immediately.

Nutritional information per serving: Kcal: 198, Protein: 9.6g, Carbs: 60.3g, Fats: 1.5g

56.   Protein Beet Greens Juice

Ingredients:

3 cups of beet greens

1 bunch of spinach

1 cup of kale, chopped

1 medium-sized artichoke head

1 large cucumber

3 tbsp of parsley, chopped

¼ tsp of Himalayan salt

Preparation:

Combine beet greens, spinach, kale and parsley in a large colander. Wash thoroughly under cold running water. Drain and roughly chop it. Set aside.

Trim off the outer wilted layers of the artichoke. Wash and cut into small pieces. Set aside.

Wash the cucumber and cut into thick slices. Set aside.

Now, combine beet greens, spinach, kale, artichoke, cucumber, and parsley in a juicer and process until juiced.

Transfer to serving glasses and stir in the salt. Add some ice and serve immediately.

Nutritional information per serving: Kcal: 151, Protein: 21.6g, Carbs: 48.2g, Fats: 2.7g

ADDITIONAL TITLES FROM THIS AUTHOR

70 Effective Meal Recipes to Prevent and Solve Being Overweight: Burn Fat Fast by Using Proper Dieting and Smart Nutrition

By Joe Correa CSN

48 Acne Solving Meal Recipes: The Fast and Natural Path to Fixing Your Acne Problems in Less Than 10 Days!

By Joe Correa CSN

41 Alzheimer's Preventing Meal Recipes: Reduce or Eliminate Your Alzheimer's Condition in 30 Days or Less!

By Joe Correa CSN

70 Effective Breast Cancer Meal Recipes: Prevent and Fight Breast Cancer with Smart Nutrition and Powerful Foods

By Joe Correa CSN

www.ingramcontent.com/pod-product-compliance
Lightning Source LLC
Chambersburg PA
CBHW051027030426
42336CB00015B/2756